URINE THERAPY

A Way To Health And Healing.

BY

JASON WALTER.

Table of Contents.

CHAPTER 1

INTRODUCTION TO URINE THERAPY.

Urine therapy among many others is one of the ancient forms of treatment for virtually all ailments one can think of that is experienced by man. It is readily available and free to get although people find it difficult to use. Urine therapy is one of the most effective medicines naturally made available for mankind without any side effects. Due to its ease of availability, and lack of possible side effect(s) make urine underrated. It lacks the appropriate publicity it deserves in today's modern world. No one is interested in advertising a free product that can be gotten easily with no negative side effects. Despite the well-known benefits of urine therapy, it remained ignored by medical practitioners with only a few medical doctors practicing treating patients with their urine.

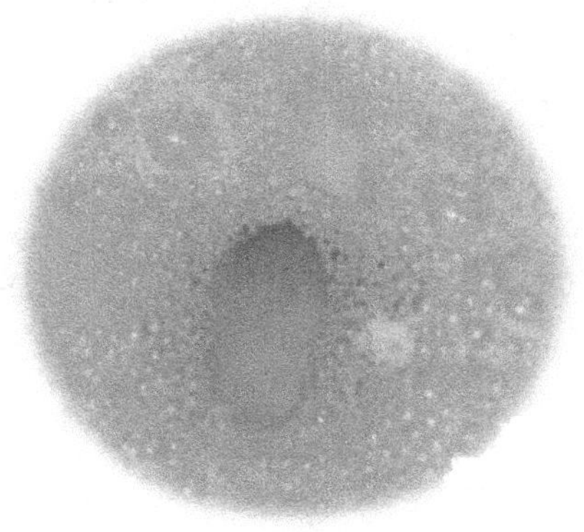

Urine therapy is among the oldest traditional medical healing methods.

Though there are several ways to heal ailments, preventing a severe ailment should be the ultimate goal. Finding the root cause of any ailment is the first step toward achieving a successful treatment plan. Treating a disease/ailment without identifying the cause is like embarking on a journey without a destination. Urine as a healing drug seems to possess answers to virtually all ailments both past, present, and future. People who witnessed the war in Jordan drank their urine with no harm experienced rather than drinking dirty polluted water.

The History of Urine.

Urine has been in use for several purposes aside from health and healing over the years. This substance is used as a form of potassium nitrate to produce gunpowder in China. The Yogis use it to improve thinking ability and reduce brainwave activities. Also, in ancient Greece, urine is used to treat some health issues such as dog bites, skin infections, general infections, scars, wounds, and even snake bites. The Romans traded urine while taxes on urine were collected by the Vespasianus. From the Russians and Celtic Druids' point of view, urine (our own urine and those from others) is used as a source of wisdom, and good health and to also sieve out toxins from our system. Urine is an all-round healing medication.

What is Urine?

Urine is simply human liquid waste produced from the kidney. The kidney is the major organ saddled with the function of filtering every substance that enters the body; retains the useful and ejects the harmful out of the body hence, it is usually advised to always drink enough water, take enough vegetables and fruits in other to ease the workload of the kidney.

Amongst many functions of the kidney is its ability to regulate the entire amount of blood that circulates the body. Therefore, the big question is "What is actually in urine that makes it a healing substance?" which will be answered in this book.

Our lifestyles are altered by so many factors ranging from diet, stress factors, social economic class, etc. in this modern day compared to the olden days. These factors make every batch of urine we produce daily a unique medicine suitable for our use at that moment. You should have a positive mindset towards its effectiveness while commencing this therapy. Urine therapy can be administered in several ways; drinking, massaging, dropping, etc. *Always ensure proper diagnoses are made by your health provider before applying any of these methods because there won't be a "cure" when the "cause" is not known.*

General Benefits of Using Urine Therapy.

Urine therapy possesses several health benefits in its usage when engaged adequately and carefully.

- Urine therapy has an incredible capacity for both chronic and acute illness.

- It is quite affordable to get, it is safe to use (with or without guidance), and very easy to practice the same time.

- The therapy can easily be practiced by anyone irrespective of age, family background, and socio-economic class.

- Unlike most modern medicine, urine therapy does not have any dangerous side effects or negative reactions.

- It is a therapy meant for every individual; both the sick and healthy. It makes the healthy individual healthier and helps the sick recover faster.

- It is the safest alternative medicine.

Despite the outstanding benefits of urine therapy, individual interest has focused mainly on modern medicine making the adoption of urine therapy quite difficult globally.

Urine therapy is an all-around medication that works for virtually all ailments. It enhances the resistance capacity of the body while improving our immune system.

<u>Urine; A Preventive Remedy.</u>

People often use medicines for the sole purpose of either curing or preventing certain ailments. However, when the body gets used to certain medications, it becomes resistant to those medications making it ineffective when needed. Therefore, living a natural life alongside healthy eating habits helps maintain health devoid of illness thus preventing ailments rather than curing them. In actual sense, urine therapy is meant to maintain our health, prevent ailments, and recycle some useful substances in the body such as enzymes, amino acids, mineral elements, and hormones but the presence of sickness in the body makes urine become a medicine for treatment.

CHAPTER 2.

METHODS OF USING URINE THERAPY.

Urine therapy is used in two methods; the internal method and the external method.

Internal Method:

♣ **Drinking:** Get some amount of urine from the middle (mid-stream) of your first-morning urine (while urinating in the morning, get some quantity after the first few drops of the flow) using a container or glass. Drink it while it's still very fresh; at least an hour before or after your first meal of the day. *Taking the* *liquid before meal (on an empty stomach) gives a better effect compared to after meal*. If the smell from the urine feels uncomfortable for you, you can as well dilute it with water or mix it with any juice of your choice.

♣ **<u>Drops:</u>** Applying some drops of urine under the tongue using an eye dropper is another method that helps determine the right dosage of urine taken while obtaining the best result. Rather than drinking a large quantity of urine at once, you can apply about 1-20 drops of urine (apply a few drops at different intervals) under the tongue. For a proper treatment pattern, take fresh urine in the morning using an eye dropper that will be taken morning (first thing before meal) and evening (last thing before bedtime);

Day 1: Apply 1-5 drops of urine under the tongue twice daily

Day 2: 5 – 10 drops twice daily

Day 3: 5 – 10 drops twice daily

The above dosage can be maintained or increased if necessary, till there is recovery from the ailment being treated.

* **Douching:** Using urine for douching helps reduce discomfort and heal vagina-related infections and diseases. You can use fresh or old urine as you so desire.

- ♣ **<u>Ear Drop</u>:** Urine can be used to treat ear infections by applying about 2-3 drops into the affected ear(s) then close the outer tip of the ear with a cotton wool so the urine doesn't spill out. Fresh urine is often used but some therapists recommend old urine particularly a 4-day-old urine because it seems more effective due to its concentration compared to fresh urine.

- ♣ **<u>Enemas</u>:** Enema is simply the injection of fluids into the body system to enhance bowel emptying. Urine therapists inject urine into the patients' system to aid bowel movement because the intestine absorbs substance better when injected compared to when given orally.

However, it is always advised to seek medical expertise help and ensure you know the right thing to do before self-medicating.

- ♣ **<u>Gargle and store in the mouth:</u>** This method may be difficult for beginners and easy for those with experience in urine therapy. Put fresh urine, store it in the mouth for about 20-30 minutes, properly gargle it in the mouth and spit it out afterward. This will help treat mouth diseases such as sore throat, toothache, bleeding gum, or even paradentosis.

- ♣ **<u>Injection method:</u>** Ensure this is carried out by a professional medical practitioner only. The urine is injected into the muscle through the skin. This is often the best option for those individuals who find it difficult to drink urine and it is usually more effective compared to the oral (drinking) method. The method is mostly carried out on patients who are unconscious by using the urine of another person of the same sex.

♣ **<u>Sniffing method</u>:** This method of urine therapy is normally used when there are issues with the eyes, nose, or even a case of sinuses. You can dilute the urine with water in a situation where you get awful reactions and the stench of the urine feels very strong.

<u>**How to use it;**</u>

- Get a fresh urine in a container,

- Put the container close to the nose,

- Close your nostril with your hand and sniff the urine with the other nostril,

- Ensure the liquid spills out through your mouth,

- Repeat the method about 3 – 4 times

- Blow out the remaining liquid from the nose afterward.

♣ <u>**Rinsing:**</u> This method is mostly used for teeth and gum infections. Get fresh urine, put it in the mouth for about 20-30 minutes, rinse the mouth with it, and spit it out afterward.

<u>**External Method.**</u>

Most persons feel comfortable using urine therapy externally compared to the internal method of usage particularly when an old urine (urine that has stayed for days) is being used because they feel the older the urine, the more effective it is. All you need do is;

- Get your fresh urine,

- Put inside a glass bottle with a cover,

- Wrap the bottle with a cloth: This will help make air circulate the bottle properly and aid adequate fermentation, giving you an alkaline effect. The fermentation process converts the urea to ammonia which makes the urine produce a very stench odor that makes it very effective.

Below are some external methods of using urine therapy;

For Baths.

- **Footbath:** Footbath with urine is the most common urine treatment for foot-related diseases, skin diseases like eczema, adequate blood circulation around the feet, and bladder-related ailments. Get fresh or old (4 days old) urine, heat it and apply it on the affected area.

- **Hip bath/sitting bath:** This is a method mostly recommended for anal or genital problems (bleeding for the anus or genital areas).

<u>How to use it:</u>

- Get enough fresh urine (you can store all the urine you produce throughout that day to be used in the evening). It can be used either hot, warm, or cold depending on your preference.
- Turn the urine into a bathtub or big bowl. You can add water to the urine to make it adequate for your use.
- Sit on the urine inside the bowl or bathtub for about 20-30 minutes.
- Repeat this procedure till the ailment heals.

- **<u>Steam Bath:</u>** Get old urine (you can mix it with water) heated up in a bowl, get a wrapper, and cover up yourself and the bowl. Ensure the steam from the hot urine touches the affected area. This is mostly used for skin infections.

- **<u>Eye Bath and Eye Drops:</u>** Most eye problems are treated with urine therapy. Get fresh urine, boil it, allow it to settle (cool) for some time, put it inside a container, use it to wash your eyes regularly and put some drops (1-2 drops) into the affected eye using a dropper.

For Compression.

- Put fresh urine in a container,

- Put the container inside hot water to warm the urine (to make the urine hot),

- Deep a rag (either a piece of cloth or a face towel),

- Place the urine-soaked towel on the affected area

- Do this till there is a positive result.

For Massages.

- **<u>Bodily Massage:</u>** Massaging the body with urine helps improve the skin outlook and aids proper circulation of blood around the body system. It is also believed that urine massage during the fasting season gives the body relevant support and adequate nourishment the body needs through the skin.

- **<u>Massages on the Hair and Scalp</u>:** Urine therapists often massage patient's head with urine for adequate scalp development and to heal certain hair and scalp-related problems such as hair loss, stunted hair growth, and even dandruff.

How to do this;

- Get fresh urine,
- Properly massage it on the patient's scalp, allow it to sit in for about 1 hour,
- Thoroughly wash the head with warm water without soap or shampoo.

- **<u>Rubbing as cream:</u>** Using urine as a form of body cream helps to generally care for the skin. Most of our body creams have urea in their content even the most expensive facial creams that we buy from beauticians. However, your urine gives you a more concentrated and balanced content needed to treat your skin compared to those contained in the facial creams we buy.

Note:

Though there haven't been any recorded cases of contrary side effects from the use of urine as an alternative medicine, some precautions need to be taken while using this therapy particularly as it relates to our diet; a major influencer on how our urine will taste as we drink our urine on a regular basis because just like taking general medicine, cases of overdose can occur in drinking urine. Though some medical experts suggest that urine therapy should not be taken alongside other modern medications while others suggest that the two medications can be taken simultaneously but in lesser dosages which can be increased and decreased on a daily basis (an increase in urine intake and a decrease in modern medicine till the modern medicine is no longer needed). In all of these, always seek medical advice for proper guidance.

CHAPTER 3.

POTENTIAL SIDE REACTIONS TO THE USE OF URINE THERAPY.

* **<u>Cough and Cold:</u>** This may occur in the respiratory passage due to the removal of mucous from the lungs.

* **<u>General body weakness:</u>** Due to the presence of excess toxins in the body. Hence, it is advised to always get adequate rest and eat proper diet while on urine therapy.

* **<u>Feverish condition:</u>** Mild fever might occur in the course of using urine therapy which often shows that the body

is burning up irrelevant toxins that are present.

* **<u>Watery stool</u>:** Having watery stool may occur after taking urine.

* **<u>Skin reactions</u>:** Some skin reactions such as pimples, rashes, or boils may occur in the course of taking urine therapy particularly within 3-7 days of taking the therapy.

* **<u>Nausea/Vomiting</u>:** This is usually the first reaction that takes place after drinking urine due to our mind's reaction to the smell of the urine. Urine actually has a very stench odor and taste maybe due to illness or other factors and drinking it might be quite difficult.

However, mixing it with water makes it easier to pass through the throat.

Vomiting while on urine therapy does not cause any danger but if it persists you can seek professional assistance, and substitute urine with other liquids for some time before drinking urine again.

* **<u>People with chronic disease:</u>** Individuals with chronic diseases like kidney problems, liver or heart disease should always consult a professional therapist before engaging in any medication.

* **<u>Pregnant women:</u>** Those in this category are advised not to drink their first-morning urine but the third urine

when they must have drank other liquids first as the first-morning urine is often too concentrated for their condition.

CHAPTER 4.

URINE AS A PREVENTATIVE THERAPY?

People often take medications for the purpose of preventing certain illnesses and one may wonder how they know the exact ailment to prevent and how certain they are of the medication's ability to prevent such ailment. Though preventing an ailment is better than curing it however, taking medications for an ailment that is not present is more like introducing an ailment than preventing one. Also constantly taking a medication when there is no illness makes the body resistant to that medication when it is needed to cure an ailment. Therefore, practicing a good healthy lifestyle including eating healthy meals provides us with all the prevention we need from ailments, not therapy/medication. Medication is only needed when there is a threat to health.

For a healthy individual, urine therapy is just a way of maintaining our health and recycling relevant substances (such hormones, minerals, amino acids, and enzymes) produced in the body while urine therapy for an unhealthy person is used as a medicine when illness develops in the body. Every illness has its antidotes and these antidotes are found in our urine.

The quality of our urine basically depends on the diet pattern. What you eat will determine how the urine you produce will be like hence it is always advised that we imbibe a good dietary pattern as this will ensure the healthiness of our bladders, kidneys and in the long run, our urinary tract. Urine changes in quality every minute with several ingredients present in its content. Therefore, when using it for treatment, you must understand which part of your diet in this substance (urine) is being recycled in the therapy. Urine is actually meant for health maintenance as such, drinking about 200ml of urine daily is a perfect dose with no harmful side effects.

However, when it comes to treating illness, one needs to be conscious of diet in other to produce healthy urine.

♣ What it is in Urine?

The reason why urine works, has been difficult to explain by scientists due to the different analysis that comes from different people's urine samples. Over the years, scientists have tried to bring out different ingredients in urine and they could only discover *urea* as a major ingredient in urine that has no negative side effects. Among several ingredients present in urine, below as some important ingredients alongside their effects on the body.

- <u>**Agglutinins and Precipitins:**</u> Agglutinin is a substance found in the blood that makes particles change from liquid form to a thick form while precipitins are reactions between antibodies and antigens. These two substances serve as a neutralizing force and are majorly used for the treatment of polio virus and other similar viruses.

- **Allantoin:** This substance is used as a moisturizing agent for the treatment and prevention of any skin-related problems. It is one of the basic ingredients in cream production. It aids in proper wound healing.

- <u>**DHEA:**</u> DHEA popularly known as Dehydroepiandrosterone/Dehydroisoand rosterone is the substance that helps to prevent diabetes, cancer of the breast, anemia; particularly plastic anemia, and obesity.

- **Gastric Secretory Depressants:** It helps prevent peptic ulcer growth.

- **Protein Globulins:** This ingredient contains different antibodies that help ward off allergies in the body.

- **Urea:** It is the antibacterial property present in urine. It acts as an oxidizing element with an organic solvent that has the ability to dissolve fats in the body alongside natural secretion capacity.

- **Uric Acid:** This controls aging and processes the presence of free radical scavengers in the body.

<u>**Dosaging in Urine Therapy.**</u>

Dosage intake in urine therapy solely depends on what you need the therapy for and the method of treatment you are using. That is if you are drinking, as a drop, bath, or massage. Just as we are different individuals, so do we have different diet patterns, react to things differently, and produce different urine daily. Therefore, the quantity of liquids (water) we take per day has the capacity to tamper with our urine concentration level.

For health maintenance and treatment of minor complaints, the following treatment/dosage pattern can be followed;

- **<u>For drinking</u>:** You can take about 200ml – 300ml of fresh urine (midstream morning urine) *except for pregnant women.*

- **<u>For Alternative therapy (urine as a homeopathic)</u>:** Place about 3 drops of urine under the tongue every hour. You can increase the time frame once you notice improvement or there's an allergic reaction (maybe apply it every 3-4 hours rather than every hour).

- **<u>As Drops</u>:** Get fresh urine, put in an eye dropper, and put a few drops under the tongue on a daily basis. You can break the treatment pattern down into days not longer than 3 days alongside the number of drops to be applied.

Day 1 – apply about 1-5 drops

Day 2 – apply 5-10 drops

Day 3 – apply 5 – 10 drops twice a day (first in the morning and last thing at night before bed).

You can either maintain this dosage pattern till the ailment is taken care of or increase it if the need arises.

CHAPTER 5.

COMMON DISEASES AND THEIR TREATMENT WITH URINE.

Below are some common diseases and their suggested treatment pattern with urine therapy.

- **Anxiety:** Drink or apply drops of fresh urine under the tongue.

- **Acne:** Wash your face with fresh early morning urine.

- **Aging:** Drink one glass of fresh urine first thing in the morning. The presence of uric acid and Dehydroepiandrosterone (DHEA) found in urine helps limit aging.

- **<u>Allergies:</u>** Engage enema therapy (insert urine into the rectum), inject urine, drink urine, or drop fresh urine under the tongue.

- **<u>Arteriosclerosis:</u>** Drink a glass of urine, apply drops of fresh urine under the tongue, and also inject or massage the body with urine.

- **<u>Anaemia:</u>** Take some dietary supplements alongside drinking urine or apply drops of fresh urine under the tongue.

- Appendicitis: Drink a glass of urine, apply drops of fresh urine under the tongue, and apply a compress of towel soaked in urine on the affected area.

- **<u>Arthritis</u>:** Apply drops of fresh urine under the tongue, drink a glass of urine, and thoroughly massage the affected area with urine compress.

- **<u>Clotted blood</u>:** Drink a glass of urine and apply drops of fresh urine under the tongue.

- **<u>Blisters</u>:** Add urine to your bathing water or carry out urine compression on the affected area.

- **<u>Asthmatic condition</u>:** Apply drops of fresh urine under the tongue, take urine injection, and engage in thorough treatment aside the condition being treated.

- **<u>Athlete's foot</u>:** engage in footbath with urine.

- **<u>Backache</u>:** Massage the entire back with urine compress.

- **<u>Cramps</u>:** Take calcium-contained meal, and massage the affected area with urine.

- **<u>Bites</u>:** Wash the spot with urine, massage the surroundings and apply urine compression.

- **<u>Bladder-related disease</u>:** Wash the genital with urine, drink a glass of urine, and apply fresh drops of urine under the tongue.

- **<u>High Blood pressure</u>:** Keenly adjust your diet pattern, drink half a glass cup of urine, or apply drops of fresh urine under the tongue.

- **<u>Low blood pressure:</u>** Drink a glass of urine and apply drops of fresh urine under the tongue.

- **<u>Bowel movement:</u>** Insert urine into the rectum, drink small quantity of urine, and apply drops of flesh urine under the tongue.

- **<u>Bleeding in the Brain:</u>** Apply urine compress on the head, drink a glass of urine, and apply drops of flesh urine under the tongue.

- **<u>Burns:</u>** Apply urine compression and massage the affected area.

- **<u>Cancer diseases:</u>** Thoroughly apply the urine to the cancer-affected area.

- **<u>Prolonged Fatigue Syndrome:</u>** Drink cold urine, gargle some quantity of urine in the mouth, you can sniff it, and also apply fresh drops of urine under the tongue.

- **<u>Constipation</u>:** Drink a glass of urine or insert urine into the rectum, and also apply fresh drops of urine under the tongue.

- **<u>Oral-related problems</u>:** Rinse the mouth with fresh urine daily; put some urine inside the mouth, hold it in for about 10-15 minutes, thoroughly gargle it in the mouth, and spit it out afterwards. Do this 3-5 times daily or as convenient for you. This will help the gum absorb the urine properly while addressing the ailment and making the loosed tooth firmer.

- **<u>Dysentery:</u>** Engage in intermediate fasting, drink a glass of urine, and apply fresh drops of urine under the tongue.

- **<u>Eczema:</u>** Massage the area with old urine and carry out urine compression on the spot.

- **<u>Eye Problem:</u>** Apply 2 drops of fresh urine to the affected eye(s) 2-3 times daily, get a cup filled with urine, allow it to settle for some time, and blink the affected eye inside the cup filled with urine. Do this for at least 3-4 days.

- **<u>Heartburn:</u>** Carefully adjust your daily diet and apply drops of fresh urine under the tongue.

- **<u>Jaundice</u>:** Drink a glass of urine, engage in intermediate fasting, and apply drops of fresh urine under the tongue

- **<u>Kidney-related ailment</u>:** Kidney treatment with urine therapy solely depends on how severe the problem is. The following treatment steps can be taken;

  - Drink half a glass of fresh urine 3 times daily and increase it to 1 – 1 ½ glass daily after 8-10 days of treatment.

  - Massage the stomach and the entire body twice daily with a 7-day-old urine.

  - Carry out compression with old urine 2-3 times daily for about 30 minutes.

- Eat less heavy meals for easy digestion.

- **<u>Meningitis</u>:** Drink a glass of urine, apply drops of fresh urine under the tongue, and carry out head compress with urine.

- **<u>Pneumonia</u>:** Apply drops of fresh urine under the tongue daily, engage in fasting, and also drink a glass of urine daily.

- **<u>Rash</u>:** Wash the affected spot with urine

- **<u>Rheumatism</u>:** Thoroughly massage the affected area with old urine, drink a glass of fresh urine, and apply drops of fresh urine under the tongue.

- **<u>Skin diseases</u>:** Carefully wash the skin with fresh urine, and carry out steam bath using old urine mixed with warm water.

- **<u>Heart disease:</u>** Drink a glass of urine once daily, massage the body with urine (personal urine or urine from another person) focusing on the face, neck, and feet; wash it out after 2 hours of massage with warm water, maintain a healthy diet for a period of one month.

- **<u>Hair loss:</u>** Daily rub the head with old urine.

Other Uses of Urine.

Throughout history, urine has been used for several reasons aside healing purposes. For instance, gunpowder is understood to be made from urine, and in recent times, it is believed that urine can remove stains from fabrics as well as skin dirt/acne with no negative side effects.

CHAPTER 6.

SUMMARY.

Summarily, urine therapy has so many benefits that we can even imagine due to its positive effects on virtually all ailments while continually maintaining our health. However, this alternative medicine hasn't gotten enough popularity in the world today. Due to the much confidence we have in modern medicine, we tend to undermine the curative ability of home-made medications. Urine therapy is a goo-to-medication in times of emergency with amazing healing capacity.

Some health issues can be prevented with urine therapy. So, rather than look for cure, we can prevent the illness from arising. Although some persons find it very difficult to administer this personally produced drug.

9 798334 892385